Anna Erenbourg

Down's syndrome decision support system for women antenatal choice

AF153278

Anna Erenbourg

Down's syndrome decision support system for women antenatal choice

LAP LAMBERT Academic Publishing

Impressum / Imprint

Bibliografische Information der Deutschen Nationalbibliothek: Die Deutsche Nationalbibliothek verzeichnet diese Publikation in der Deutschen Nationalbibliografie; detaillierte bibliografische Daten sind im Internet über http://dnb.d-nb.de abrufbar.

Alle in diesem Buch genannten Marken und Produktnamen unterliegen warenzeichen-, marken- oder patentrechtlichem Schutz bzw. sind Warenzeichen oder eingetragene Warenzeichen der jeweiligen Inhaber. Die Wiedergabe von Marken, Produktnamen, Gebrauchsnamen, Handelsnamen, Warenbezeichnungen u.s.w. in diesem Werk berechtigt auch ohne besondere Kennzeichnung nicht zu der Annahme, dass solche Namen im Sinne der Warenzeichen- und Markenschutzgesetzgebung als frei zu betrachten wären und daher von jedermann benutzt werden dürften.

Bibliographic information published by the Deutsche Nationalbibliothek: The Deutsche Nationalbibliothek lists this publication in the Deutsche Nationalbibliografie; detailed bibliographic data are available in the Internet at http://dnb.d-nb.de.

Any brand names and product names mentioned in this book are subject to trademark, brand or patent protection and are trademarks or registered trademarks of their respective holders. The use of brand names, product names, common names, trade names, product descriptions etc. even without a particular marking in this works is in no way to be construed to mean that such names may be regarded as unrestricted in respect of trademark and brand protection legislation and could thus be used by anyone.

Coverbild / Cover image: www.ingimage.com

Verlag / Publisher:
LAP LAMBERT Academic Publishing
ist ein Imprint der / is a trademark of
OmniScriptum GmbH & Co. KG
Heinrich-Böcking-Str. 6-8, 66121 Saarbrücken, Deutschland / Germany
Email: info@lap-publishing.com

Herstellung: siehe letzte Seite /
Printed at: see last page
ISBN: 978-3-659-50321-4

Zugl. / Approved by: London, University of London, Dissertation, 2008

Acknowledgements

I would like to express my gratitude to my family who always supported me and to the co-authors of this book Professor Judith Stephenson, Mr Pran Pandya, Professor Jack Dowie and Miss Tricia Jones.

Contents

Chapter 1: Introduction

Down's syndrome (DS) is one of the commonest chromosomal abnormalities, affecting 6 births per thousand in the UK. Although increased maternal age is a strong risk factor, most DS babies are born to younger women at low individual risk because many more pregnancies occur in women under 35 years (Stone DH et al., 1989).

A wide range of biochemical tests, plus measurements taken during antenatal ultrasound have been developed to assess DS risk more accurately than maternal age alone (Haddow et al, 1994; Benn, 2003).

These are routinely used in clinical practice as non-invasive screening tests (Copel et al, 1999). A summary of different screening options offered and performance characteristics of different tests is available in Table 1.

In the UK every pregnant woman should be given information about the baby's development during pregnancy, nutrition diet and exercise, the pregnancy care pathway[1] and place of birth, mental health issues, breastfeeding workshops, antenatal classes participation and ANC (antenatal care) screenings by 10 weeks of gestational age (GA) (NCC-WCH, 2008).

To deliver this information, women should be told, at their first contact with health professionals (HP), to book an antenatal discussion at around 8 weeks of pregnancy at hospitals, GP practices or community midwives units.

During the visit HP should introduce women to different available screening tests offered in pregnancy. Information about DS screening would be included in this discussion as part of screening for fetal anomalies.

Pregnant women are initially offered a screening test for DS on the understanding that there is a future possibility that they will require a further diagnostic test if the result shows them at high risk (NCC-WCH, 2008).

After a woman has undertaken one of the available screening tests they are given results, estimating their individual probability of giving birth to a DS baby. This probability is calculated by the combination of maternal age at expected delivery date (EDD), different biochemical markers and ultrasound findings, depending on the kind of test chosen (Table 1).

---

[1] See Figure 1: Pregnancy care pathway in the UK.

In the case of a positive test suggesting a woman was at higher risk for having a baby with Down's, she would be offered an invasive procedure, either amniocentesis or chorionic villous sampling (CVS), depending on gestational age.

The woman could decide to proceed with further investigations or opt out of further testing. The risks of miscarriage related to invasive procedures are 1% for amniocentesis and 3% related to CVS (RCOG, 2005). If a woman proceed to diagnostic testing and confirmatory abnormalities were identified, she would be offered a termination of pregnancy (TOP).

In UCLH, where this study was carried out, the screening test offered is the integrated. This is the test of choice, in terms of efficacy, safety and cost, based on findings of the SURUSS study (Wald et al, 2003).

In case a patient accesses the service in the second trimester of pregnancy, too late to undertake integrated, she will be offered a quadruple test. Other tests are routinely used by referrals or if a single patient expresses her preference for another specific screening test.

Even if a patient desires to undertake a diagnostic option, she should still undertake a screening test first and then decide whether going further after results. There is a disparity of tests on offer all over the UK, so not every Trust will offer the entire spectrum of tests available, depending mainly on sonographers, skilled to perform ultrasound scans.

Figure 1: Pregnancy care pathway in the UK.

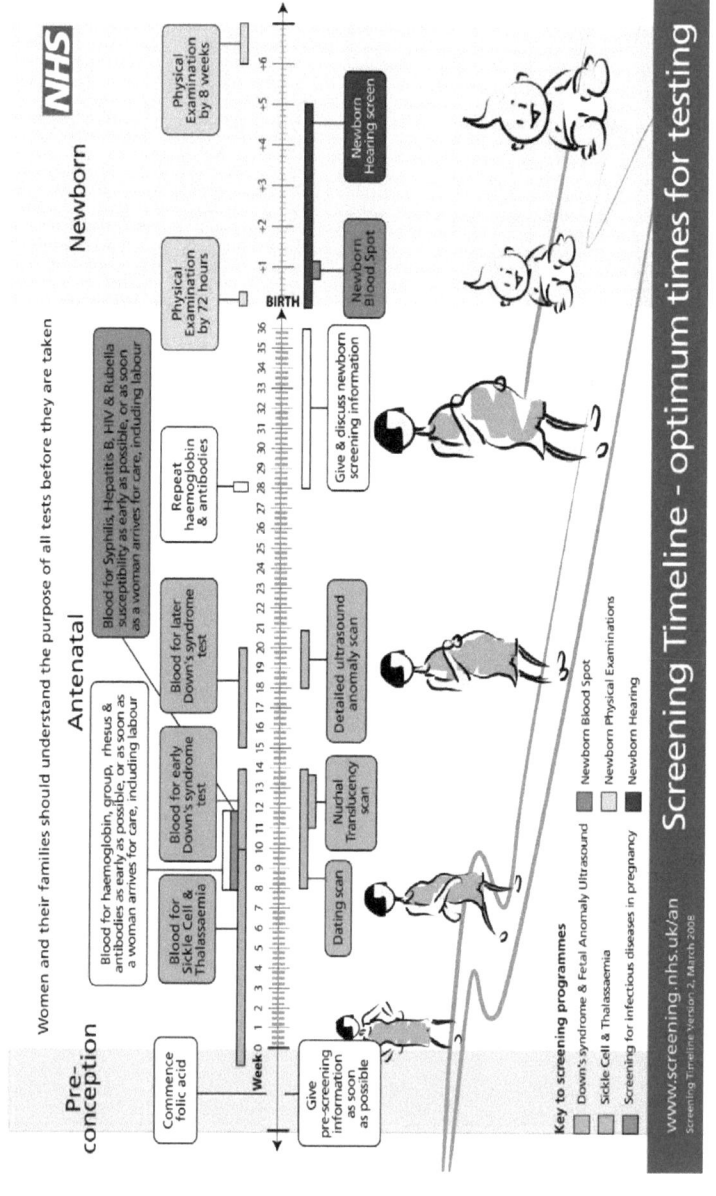

Table 1: Down's syndrome Screening Tests

Tests' Characteristics / Screening Options	Gestational Age		Tests' Performance DR (%) = 85%	
	11-14 weeks	15-20 weeks	FPR (%) (False Positive Rate)	N° DS pregnancies detected for each procedure-related unaffected fetal loss
Combined	NT, β-hCG, PAPP-A	-	6.1	3.9
Double	-	β-hCG, uE3	13.1	1.8
Triple	-	β-hCG, uE3, AFP	9.3	2.6
Quadruple	-	β-hCG, uE3, AFP, inhibin A	6.2	3.8
Integrated	Combined	uE3, AFP, inhibin A	1.2	19.2
Serum Integrated	PAPP-A, β-hCG	UE3, AFP, inhibin A	2.7	9.1

Note: All tests include maternal age and free β-hCG is used rather than total hCG. The first trimester markers PAPP-A and free β-hCG are based on the median in DS pregnancies at 10 completed weeks and the NT SD in unaffected pregnancies is applicable to 10 completed weeks. Number of DS detected is obtained dividing number of procedure related unaffected fetal losses in 100,000 women screened (80% uptake rate for Amniocentesis or CVS and 0.9% fetal loss rate attributable to the procedure) by the number of DS pregnancies detected (assuming 90% uptake rate for Amniocentesis and CVS because women with affected pregnancies tend to have higher risk and so are more likely to accept diagnostic testing).
This table has been partially reproduced from SURUSS, Wald at al., 2003.

The body of literature regarding psychosocial aspects of DS Prenatal screening is extremely rich and complex. Following the introduction of serum screening for DS, clinicians' concerns initially focused on anxiety relating to the screening process. Following this interest shifted to quantifying women's knowledge and understanding of the available options, and how to improve their awareness in order that they could make an informed decision (Green JM et al., 2004).

Some women in fact find hard to interpret information about risk or to appreciate the distinction between screening and diagnostic results (Hall et al, 2000). Another complexity for women contemplating DS screening or diagnosis, is timing. Different screening tests must be done at specific stages of pregnancy and the psychological consequences of termination following a positive diagnosis of DS are clearly affected by the stage of pregnancy (Hall et al, 2000).

Latterly much research work has been directed towards assessing the reasons why women decide to be tested for DS and to explore social and ethnic inequalities in either offer or uptake of screening (Rowe RE et al., 2003).

Attention has also been drawn more recently to assessing whether women are making truly informed decisions, evaluating the impact of awareness on screening uptake and anxiety levels and to understand the actual decision-making process (Green JM et al., 2004). But do women take informed decisions about prenatal screening and how do they take them? An informed choice has been defined as:

A reasoned choice which is made by a reasonable individual using relevant information about possible advantages and disadvantages of all possible courses of action, in accord with individual belief (Bekker H et al., 1999).

In most past work inappropriate methods have been used in the assessment of informed choice. The multidimensionality of the concept has been largely neglected (Marteau et al., 2001; Gorounti K et al., 2008) and unreliable self-report methods have been used for assessment (Green JM et al., 2004).

However, despite these criticisms, a recent review evaluated different aspects of informed choice making. These aspects included awareness of relevant information, appropriate perception of own individual risk, processing capacity, stability in own values over time, satisfaction with decision taken and perceived decisional conflict (Green JM et al., 2004).

The researchers identified a gap between women's desire to make an informed choice about screening and their awareness and skills to achieve it. These conclusions would support the hypothesis that prescriptive theory could best explain prenatal decision-making. This theory suggests that humans are limited in their processing capacity by nature. Because of this, individuals would be naturally poor decision-makers unless helped by aiding tools to support them through the decision-making process (Bekker H et al, 1999).

Different decision-making models have been applied to assist making health decisions that involve risk. One of the most commonly mentioned is subjective expected utilities theory (SEU). This assumes that individuals should make decisions through balancing the likelihood of the outcomes occurring and their own values and beliefs (Bekker HL et al, 2004).

As previously considered, although models based on SEU would offer a valid rigorous scientific method to represent women's decisions, they would imply a rational way of thinking not entirely representative of the way prenatal choices are taken in reality. In fact, the role of emotions in decision-making is increasingly recognized and in recent studies the emotional contribution in response to risky situations has been affirmed (Van den Berg M et al., 2008).

A development of SEU models that conserves the main principles of SEU theory, but allows for more flexibility and adaptability is Multi-criteria decision models (MCDM). In these models, weights provided by users don't meet all formal criteria for being classical subjective expected utilities. This loss in rigor is the trade off for including other dimensions of decision-making over an above rationality, such as emotions and attitudes towards specific outcomes.

To help women make informed choices about DS screening or diagnosis, this study set out to develop a DSS based on decision analysis. Essentially this is a method for breaking down complex problems or questions into manageable components, and then combining them logically to show the best course of action (French et al, 2007).

The model will combine individual values (e.g. the undesirability attached to miscarriage associated with diagnostic test) with epidemiological data relevant to the different interventions (e.g. the probability of miscarriage following diagnostic tests).

The model sets out to combine the best available scientific evidence with quantitative assessments of the individual user's preference and values. Annalisa, the software that was used to develop the DSS is a MCDM. This DSS will consent users to express preferences about their concerns using a visual analogue scale, giving them in response the best course of actions on the base of given preferences[2].

---

[2] See Figure 2: DSS Annalisa & Down's syndrome Prenatal Choice

Chapter 2: Methods

Ethical approval was obtained both from UCL/UCLH Committee and LSHTM. To identify the factors involved in the decision-making process about antenatal DS screening, focus groups were initially felt to be the optimal method. These would have had the advantage of being a cheap, quick and reliable method of collecting information and the interaction among participants could have helped in eliciting concerns in the decision-making.

However despite these benefits, the practicality of asking women to come back for a second time to participate was too inconvenient, leading to difficulties in the recruitment phase. The initial protocol was therefore amended and face-to-face interviews were conducted instead, as the preferred data collection method. Twenty semi-structured interviews were carried out to collect similar information from a variety of women and the original topic guide was adapted and extended to fulfill the new method requirements[3].

To include a wide variety of opinions women were initially selected by parity and maternal age. The hypothesis was that the decision-making process could have been affected by previous antenatal experiences since attitudes might change after experiencing pregnancy and childbirth (Etchegary et al., 2008).

Because of its impact on the risk of conceiving a Down's child, maternal age was considered another important factor to take into account in selecting women. Older women's (35+ yrs) decision process could have differed from young mothers (under 35 yrs), since both nulliparity and prior pregnancies have been recognized as powerful factors affecting decisions (Etchegary et al., 2008). For ethical reasons women diagnosed a Down baby in previous pregnancies were excluded to avoid possible psychological consequences due to recalling events.

Women accessing UCLH antenatal care service for a 20-weeks scan were recruited accordingly to parity and age. Women are routinely offered a scan at this GA.

---

[3] See Figure 3: Down's syndrome Topics Guide.

Figure 3: Down's syndrome original Topics Guide.

Down's Syndrome Topics Guide

1. What experiences have you had in relation to screening or diagnosis of Down's syndrome in pregnancy?

- Is this the first time that you have been screened
- Is it your first pregnancy
- Why did you decide to be tested for Down's syndrome
- Have you thought about termination
- Is it an age related decision
- Have you been influenced by the fact that it's not your first pregnancy

2. What options were available to you?

- Did you decide for a screening or a diagnostic test and why
- Are you aware of the difference between a screening and a diagnostic test
- Have you asked the rate of success in estimating the risk
- Have you asked which are the possible complications related to every specific technique
- Early 13 weeks/Late 16 weeks
- Screening/Diagnostic
- Screening: Combined/Integrated
- Diagnostic: Amnio/CVS

3. How easy or difficult was it to reach a decision on screening/diagnosis options?

- Do you think you have received a reasonable amount of information
- Where did you get this information from (information sheet, internet, midwife, friends ...)
- Why do you think that the decision has been difficult (emotional reasons/ethical reasons, a lot of different possibilities, lack of information.)

4. What information were you given, before reaching a decision about screening/diagnosis?

- How to interpret the results (in term of Risk/Probability/and High/Low risk categories
- Complications/risk miscarriage
- Would you be happy receiving a result in terms of risk

5. What information did you want before reaching a decision about screening/diagnosis?

- What do you consider have been helpful, unhelpful, clear, unclear, confusing, alarming

6. What factors influenced you more in reaching a decision?

- Other people opinion, ethical, religious
- Do you think that you have been influenced in taking the decision
- By whom (partner, doctor, midwife, friends' opinion...)

7. How do you think this aspect of antenatal care should be handled in future?

- Something that should have been done better
- Do you think that a support system would be helpful
- Do you think that an information package would be helpful
- Any other comments

Furthermore 20 weeks is also the deadline for the second appointment of the Integrated Test, so by then each woman would have already taken her decision. This would avoid the study influencing participants in their decision-making. Potential participants were approached, informed about the study aims and methods and a consent form was given if they wanted to take part.

The first 5 interviews were carried out at the beginning of 2007 at UCLH ultrasound department and interviewees had already undertaken the integrated test. Interviews were recorded and transcribed. The analytic process started during transcription of the first set of interviews through familiarisation and a rudimentary coding procedure. The main points of discussion were obviously in harmony with themes proposed by the topics guide3.

To analyze this data, some of the principles of Grounded Theory were applied. These were mainly constant comparison and deviant cases identification. Because the methods of data collection, the inclusion criteria and topics of discussion were all redefined on the basis of emerging information, principles of Grounded theory were thought to be the best method of analysis due to its maximum flexibility.

Recruitment criteria were refined on the basis of the findings from transcribing the first interviews. Women opting for either Combined, other screening or Diagnostic tests were included since they were felt to be an important source of key knowledge that would otherwise have been lost. The initial Topic guide was modified with further questions about possible factors affecting decision-making process, information given before taking the decision and why in case of doubts they wouldn't ask for more details about tests.

Following the modifications to the data collection, the subsequent interviews were recorded, transcribed and analysed. Demographic data and the reproductive history of each woman were collected from patients' records (Table 2). Out of twenty women interviewed their partners accompanied fifteen. Since most of the couples took the decision together they expressed a willingness to participate jointly in the discussion and it was decided to respect their choice.

Table 2: Demographic & Reproductive characteristics of the sample.

Maternal age	
Mean	36.7 yrs
Range	21-44 yrs
	N° women
Parity	
Multiparous	12
Nulliparous	8

	20
Down's Test (at current pregnancy)	
Screening	
Triple	1
Quadruple	1
Integrated	9
Combined	5
Diagnostic	
CVS	2
Amniocentesis	2

	20
Previous Miscarriage	
Yes	6
No	13
Recurrent	1

	20
Way of accessing service	
GP practice	3
Community Midwife	1
Referral by other Hospital	5
UCLH Antenatal discussion	11

	20

Note: Women going for invasive testing were all offered and undertook also a screening test following NICE guidelines. NICE suggests that all women should be offered a screening test first, despite their intentions of undertaking an invasive procedure. Women were included in the category relative to last test undertaken.

14

To enhance reliability coded fragments of text were constantly compared and a headings and subheadings scheme was generated[4]. The analysis was carried out first on transcripts brainstorming key themes, and then using N-vivo to support constant comparison technique and charting phase.

During the charting phase the main subheadings were identified and emerging themes such as what it would mean to women having a DS child and what women think about NHS services came up through the inductive process.

Main patterns were mapped; deviant cases and emerging ideas were recognised mainly among women choosing a diagnostic option, enriching our pool of data. The Interviewing and analysing process was interrupted when we judged that saturation was reached.

We constructed a preliminary DSS and input empirical data that would underlie it (e.g. risk of miscarriage following invasive procedure).

The empirical data is derived from published literature on the probabilities of relevant outcomes e.g. risk of miscarriage of DS and non DS fetuses at different stages of pregnancy or following diagnostic procedures, and on performance characteristics (sensitivity and specificity) of different screening tests.

Having elicited the attributes through interviews[5], they were incorporated into the decision analysis model and developed the computer interface to finalize the DSS[6].

The last stage of the project will involve testing the model interface and piloting the DSS, initially with 10 midwives and obstetricians and then with 10 women from gynecology outpatients.

The purpose here is to identify presentational aspects of the DSS that might increase concern or confusion among users. Feedback obtained will be used to refine the DSS, before further evaluation in a RCT. This dissertation will focus on the first qualitative stage of the project, presenting main results of descriptive analysis.

---

[4] See Figure 4: Down's syndrome Qualitative Analysis & N-vivo headings and subheadings scheme.
[5] See Figure 5: Results of this first stage were presented at the Annual Meeting of Institute for Women's Health, Poster Presentation.
[6] See Figure 2: DSS Annalisa & Down's syndrome Prenatal Choice

Figure 4: Down's syndrome Qualitative Analysis: N-vivo headings & subheadings scheme.

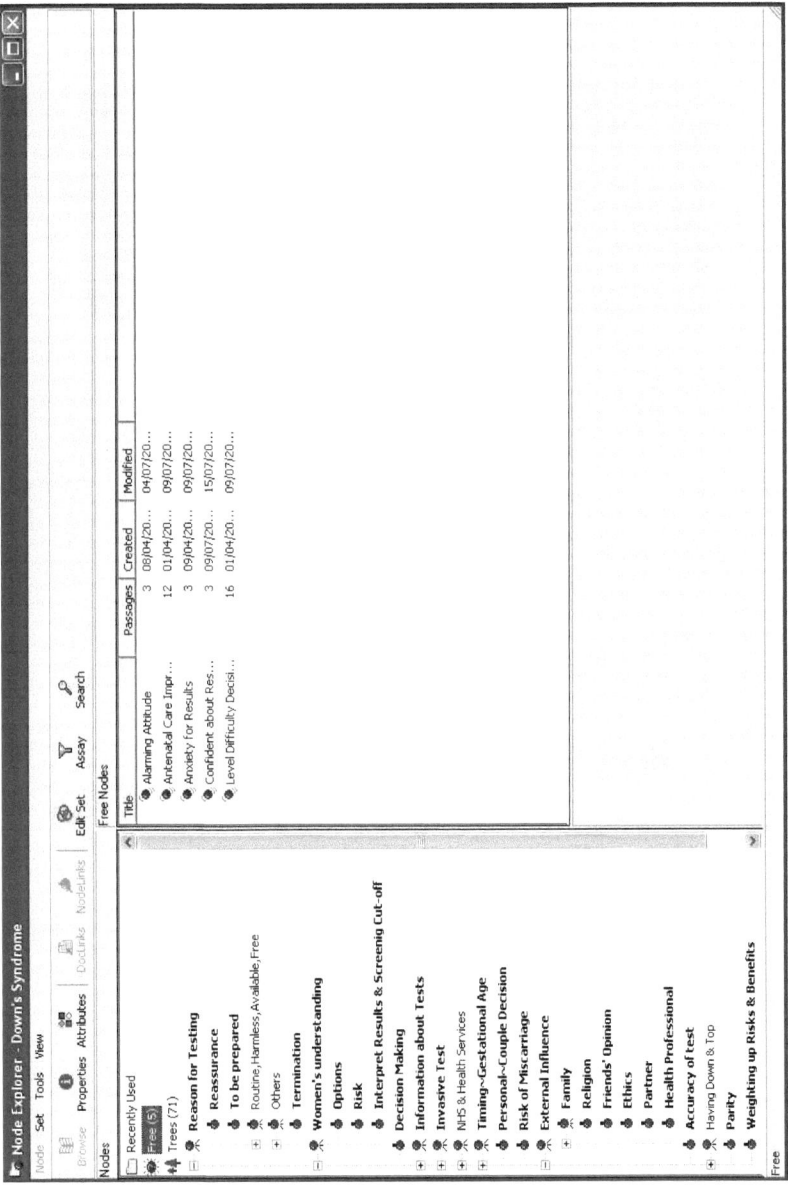

Figure 5: Poster Presentation at Annual Conference of IFWH 2007.

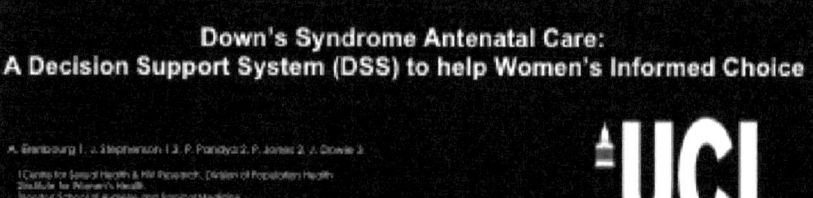

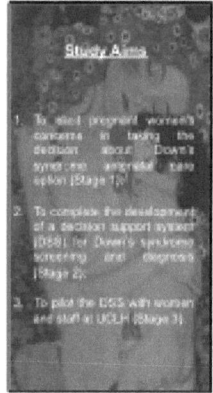

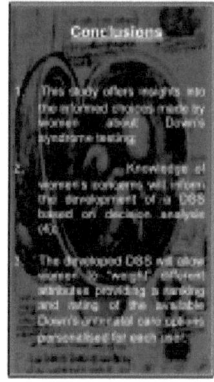

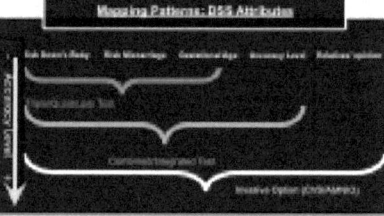

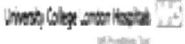

Chapter 3: Results

All women seemed to be very keen in ascertaining baby's wellbeing and didn't find the decision of getting screened very difficult. Screening is in fact correctly considered as an available, free and harmless option that women are offered. When women were asked their reasons for testing, some of them answered that they considered screening as part of a **routine**. They had been through it in previous pregnancies and they follow the offered pathway as something sensible to do, in some cases without thinking of the possible next steps.

"I've treated every pregnancy the same so with the same routine... I found that I'm pregnant, I went for all the blood testing, as well as Down's syndrome…" (Multiparous, 32 yrs)

A variety of different answers were given, some of them more recurrent. Most interviewees stated that they decided to get tested for DS for **reassurance**, or to be prepared or because they would terminate in case of DS baby. The first group of pregnant women was mainly made up of individuals who were assuming to receive a low risk result. For different reasons such as healthy lifestyle, previous negative results or young age these women feel confident about negativity of results and they wouldn't expect to receive "bad news".

"…I think we are just a little bit more confident…may be I shouldn't be but…I think I'm more confident the second time around…because it turned out so well…and then I thought I'm a very healthy person…" (Multiparous, 39yrs)

The second very common given answer was "**to be prepared**" for any problems. These women didn't feel certain about the possible outcome of testing and most of the time they preferred to postpone any alarming thoughts to post results moment.

"In a way it's to feel secure and on the other hand if there is something that it's better to detect earlier and find solutions or prepare yourself for whatever is there so…" (Multiparous, 29 yrs)

Last most quoted reason to be tested was **to terminate** in case of DS pregnancy. Women belonging to this category were generally more aware of their possible reactions and decisions in case of positive results. They decided to be tested to find out if further testing and actions had to be taken.

"R: ...ehm...basically because we have agreed as a couple that it wouldn't be in our best interest or we would find in our best interest if we had a DS child...

I: Have you ever thought of an eventual TOP?

R: That... oh yes... that would be the result if anything didn't work..." *(Multiparous, 43 yrs)*

Deviant cases from these main patterns were identified: older age, family history of DS and obeying of doctors' suggestion were given by these outliers, as main reasons to undertake screening.

If the decision of assessing baby's wellbeing through a screening test was described by women as easy, the variety of options and sometimes lack of communication were identified as the main reasons why **choosing a specific test** could be difficult. Among women expressing lack of communication and information as a cause of these difficulties, we explored reasons why they didn't ask more questions to HP. They justified it saying that they were worried. Such a distress related to testing would prevent them asking for clarifications.

Among identified difficulties in taking decisions, women mentioned lack of understanding. The majority of women had clear ideas of the distinction between screening and invasive procedures and they mentioned risk of miscarriage attached to diagnostic. Less clear was the difference between various tests: most women struggled at describing available alternatives belonging to the two categories. The other identified problem was interpreting results and the validity of the screening cut-off.

"I think I do understand the concept very well...may be I can imagine that some people might not understand the concept of risk...but when they said that 1 in 150 is high risk and 1 in 160 is low risk...that is ridiculous...that is absolutely ridiculous...especially when you think that it could be 1 in 50000... [...] ... That just doesn't seem to make sense..." *(Nulliparous, 29 yrs)*

The other difficult and painful choice was the decision among women having had a screening test and deciding to **undertake an invasive** procedure. As already mentioned many women go ahead for screening without considering the possibility of getting a high-risk result and without making decisions about diagnostic tests and TOP. This results in a kind of emotional shock at first and at that point they are forced to decide in few days whether to take the risk of miscarriage related to an invasive test or not.

"Yea…it was difficult…it was really difficult…I've been thinking of it for a very long time…and then when I came here at the second floor I was here for hours…you know…hours…worrying about having it done or not…" (Multiparous, 38 yrs)

Depending on women's intentions and attitudes towards testing, their level of knowledge and awareness in decision-making varied a lot. Some women were following a predetermined pathway without really going through a decision-making process, other were much more conscious and looking for information to take an informed decision. At the very extreme end of the spectrum, a future mother who identified, in looking for information and making decisions, the first responsibility as a mother:

" ...So you know at the end of the day it's up to me...you know...I'm the mother we are the parents and at the end of the day it's worth to do some research...what happens...what scientifically happens to my body...I thought I have a personal responsibility to this baby to make sure that...what's happening to my body and what's being...you know...it's done to me...or what's going on you know...people would tell me staff but I will read it..." (Nulliparous, 40 yrs)

Another important aspect to consider is that even among well informed women, some would postpone any decisions about invasive and TOP until after the screening period, even among women aware of diagnostic tests characteristics.

"I: ...But have you already thought of eventually going for further investigations or not...I mean is it something in your mind or...

R: ...not really we are taking a step at time...and when the result come back we will take a decision but..." (Multiparous, 35 yrs)

Independently on knowledge demand at a screening stage, necessity for information increased at the diagnostic one. Among women aiming to make an informed decision, the process was described as a weighing up, evaluating pros and cons of different strategies.

"It was weighing up...it was weighing up the possibility, the kind of risk...the risk of the procedure with the social relief that everything was going to be ok..." (Multiparous, 38 yrs)

The weighting up process involved a number of different factors, from personal perception of what having a DS baby would mean, to ethical and religious principles against abortion versus a personal attitude towards TOP. Apart from the already mentioned key factors, other important elements involved in decision-making were related to test features such as gestation at testing, risk of miscarriage and accuracy of results. Taking a decision among different options of being screened or diagnose for DS could be for some women a private decision or be influenced by external characters as family, friends and HP.

One relevant aspect to be taken into account in understanding women's decision-making is whether they consider it a **private matter** or they listen to others' ideas. A variety of opinions were expressed and among women there was a clear disagreement. Around half of interviewees thought that the decision about DS testing was pretty much private in which they automatically included their **partner** who was considered as directly and naturally involved in their choice.

"I: Right...but do you think you have been influenced by your GP's opinion or someone else's opinion?

R: No...not at all...I think it is very much personal...so it was me and my partner..." (Multiparous, 43 yrs)

Partner's role was not only supportive but actively influencing decision-making. Moreover one of the interviewee reported difficulties in absorbing information given by her HP because of the stressful situation. In that occasion she very much appreciated the presence of her husband, who could have replaced her in memorizing information.

" ...Because you are a little bit in shock you can't always register so much...and so it's quite useful for me I can have my husband here...because he absorbs what I can't, I can't absorb...and I mean in a way my brain switches off...because I'm...you know...I'm responding at a certain emotional level..." (Multiparous, 41yrs)

The other half of women showed an interest in listening to other people. The main characters playing such a role were family, friends and HP. **Family** was in some circumstances considered as a good source of emotional support or to help in information seeking. In fact almost all women used as principal sources of information antenatal discussion and NHS booklet given by HP on that occasion.

This source was not exclusive though and interviewees reported using other sources, such as pregnancy books and web resources. Websites were reported as the most common and useful source in case of insecurity. In this search, some women found help in their partner, family or friends. In particular **friends** who have experienced prenatal screening or were pregnant at the same time were occasionally identified as a great supporting network because they were sensitive and emotionally involved.

"R: ...I had a friend who was pregnant with...the same time as me the other year and we were going through the same thing and her results were...her ratio was a lot lower than mine so her risk was higher and she went on and she had the invasive test...because also she was carrying twins and they were identical...so we sort of talked about it so I think from my friends' network I've got close females I could chat with...

I: ...a kind of support...

R: ...yea...yea...and it's the kind of idea that you can't really do with your partner because they can see a bit more black or white...and girls like to have a little chat about things..." (Multiparous, 43yrs)

As this woman mentioned, having friends also pregnant, was considered probably the best partner of discussion on this matter. Sometimes women mentioned how their parents were willing to help, but intergenerational differences and the frequent changes in scientific assessment of DS risk wouldn't allow them to offer an evidence based opinion. Friends having been through DS screening offered updated knowledge as well as the same emotional involvement to be considered an empathetic point of reference for discussion.

The other important people involved were **health professionals**. For some women with previous negative experiences or with a general lack of trust in HP, the decision wouldn't involve them and their role would be restricted to inform about different possibilities in a neutral, non-judgmental way. Other women felt that a professional opinion was required and were looking forward to listen to suggestions about what to do.

Since they didn't feel comfortable in taking the decision themselves, they expressed gratitude for professional advice and human support. Moreover some women felt more secure if they could contact HP at any time in case of any doubts about options or results and if they needed emotional support and they proposed setting up a phone helpline as a possible service improvement.

The aim of this study was to elicit and identify main women's concerns in their decision-making to inform the development of a DSS. It wasn't really our intention to explore what **having a DS baby** meant to women going for a test, but obviously it was a crucial concern, which is why it came up automatically as an emerging theme during interviews. Having a child with disabilities was interpreted as a big commitment and responsibility that most of the interviewed women or couple wouldn't consider taking on.

"...And DS kids are generally quite happy...I mean not that I'm really experienced, but for what I've seen...they bring that joy and all sort of things...they are generally quite happy...except for the seek of care...but in terms of my life, and our life and the people who are already in our life...I think I just wouldn't want to go through that...I think there is a lot of hardship and a lot of responsibility..." (Multiparous, 41 yrs)

Some women answered that having a DS child would lead to such a big change in existing lifestyle, both for the parents and other children that they were not prepared to take on. Some women intimated that TOP in cases of DS was a way of protecting preexisting family from such a big change and commitment, and from the huge impact that a baby with disabilities would have on their entire lives.

"...And having a child with needs...a special needs child especially quite a severe special needs child would just have such a big effect on all of us so I don't think we could actually...it's not just me and my husband's life that we are affecting but our family and we both work long hours as well so...[...]...I think you are probably selfish from this point of view because you think of your current family rather than the potential new baby...so it's probably not thinking of their wellbeing...it's more the sort of existing people and the effect that it would have..." (Multiparous, 43 yrs)

One woman recognized as the main reason for her eventual **termination of pregnancy** (Top), the incapability of coping with a baby with handicaps. She didn't explicitly specify she meant the psychological burden of having a DS baby, but the feeling during her interview was that she was referring to that. We couldn't explore further for ethical reasons, since this woman was diagnosed a genetic anomaly in her previous pregnancy.

On the other hand there were women considering termination as the only solution in the case of DS, to prevent having to bring up a disabled child in this difficult world. Some women thought that the baby would have problems, i.e. physical. A few were worried that once they had died the child would have been alone, without anyone to take care of him/her. In this case women were not considering TOP to protect preexisting family, but in a way "to protect" the potential child from a very difficult life.

"...Well yes...before I got pregnant I thought I would definitely terminated the pregnancy if there was anything wrong...because I always think it's not about me not being happy it's about if I die who is going to take care of the baby...you know...so I think in my mind is very clear about that...[...]...you know...bring a child to the world with severe handicaps...and you know you die in your seventies and who...who is going to take care of the child..." (Multiparous, 39yrs)

Relating to this subject, women talked about TOP and expressed interesting comments about timing of termination and people' judgments towards abortion were mentioned.

"...If I had to terminate it...I don't know...I can't remember what I was going to say...I don't know if I would have done...but everybody knew I was pregnant and I would have wanted to pretend that it was a miscarriage...I wouldn't wanted to admit...[...]...but anyway I was worried about other's people' opinions..." (Multiparous, 38 yrs)

Concerns related to a second trimester versus first trimester TOP were identified. Reasons why women were more worried about a second trimester TOP were mainly due to the stronger attachment to their baby at that stage and to a wider circle of people being aware of the pregnancy and having expectations, especially relatives.

"In the back of my mind if it was negative I still...then I would...I would have terminated it either...I mean obviously we would have made the decision together if it was negative but I would have found very hard to make a decision if...you know... to terminate...because I had already seen it on the screen and seen his heart beating and it was at 6 weeks, wasn't it? And you know it was already a little baby..." (Nulliparous, 40 yrs)

As it was with termination concerns, **gestational age** was identified as an issue affecting prenatal decision. The already mentioned concerns about late TOP have consequently an impact on screening and antenatal discussion. Few women mentioned how having first contact and discussion very early in pregnancy would accelerate the entire process of searching for knowledge, screening and eventual further decisions.

Other women concentrated their interest more on the timing of screening: early option would increase the available time to make further decisions in case of positive results. One of the interviewees mentioned her concerns about late testing in relation to her right to terminate at that GA.

"…It's just thinking what if that…the results are positive and I was at high risk what other options did I have? Did I have the right to terminate? Did I have any other solutions that…do I really have to give it birth…it's just…what if something positive or high risk…what options did I have I don't know…" (Nulliparous, 34 yrs)

The general feeling was that early screening and results are desirable, so that parents would have time to speak to family, friends, doctors and decide about further testing and then eventually about TOP. Although when women were explicitly asked to weigh GA at tests/results and accuracy level, they argued that more accurate results even getting them late would be preferable.

Other concerns affecting decision-making were either related to some tests' characteristics or randomly mentioned during interviews and presumably in the back of their minds during decision processes. Tests characteristics that were identified as relevant were risk of miscarriage, physical/emotional discomfort related to invasive tests, and accuracy of different strategies.

Most women correctly mentioned **risk of miscarriage** as a possible consequence of diagnostic testing. Some of them illustrated how this risk was the reason why they chose a screening test despite the uncertainty of results. A couple of interviewees talked about their difficulties in conceiving a baby and their history of previous spontaneous miscarriages. They mentioned how the risk attached to invasive testing was absolutely unacceptable for them because of their reproductive history.

"…Yes…because I have quite an high tendency to miscarry…this has probably been the only test I would…I've been considering I think…if the results were borderline after today then I might have had a serious conversation with my gynaecologist about whether I had a more invasive test…because hen the risk for me would go up quite a lot…so that's why I'm not even thinking of it that much…" (Multiparous, 43 yrs)

Furthermore one of the interviewees mentioned that her decision was influenced by the fact that level of risk attached to an invasive test is executor-dependent.

"I didn't want to take the risk and I know that the one percent depends on where it has been done…and when I went to the US I went to the Montana were they invented it you know…so I knew that the person doing it…so I knew that the chances were much less than one percent…" (Multiparous, 39 yrs)

Women who undertook an invasive test underlined how a physical and emotional discomfort characterized the test's execution. Other women going for screening didn't mention it, so **test's discomfort and stress** of a test could be an attribute affecting the decision only in women who have experienced the invasive procedure.

Physical feeling was described as awful and invasive and quite long in terms of performing time. Moreover this physical discomfort was accompanied by a partially unexpected deep emotional involvement:

"…I spoke to a friend and she said It's fine, it's nothing you know…if it was very dangerous they wouldn't let you have it done you know…It's nothing…so I thought…It was just a kind of like…It's nothing…you know…It's like having a kind of manicure you know…I thought it was a kind of insignificant…but it's not…it's a big thing…" (Multiparous, 38 yrs)

Another important aspect mentioned exclusively by women undertaking a diagnostic option was concern about people's **judgment** on women taking the risk of an invasive procedure. This concern was expressed, but if and how effectively it affected decision-making was unclear.

"…and also I think I was worried about what people would think…I was worried that people would be a sort of judgmental about it and say well what's the point of knowing if you are not going to have a miscarriage…an abortion…" (Multiparous, 38 yrs)

Another characteristic discussed as a potential factor influencing the decision-making process was the **accuracy and uncertainty** that remains even after screening. Few women had enough knowledge and understanding of different options to comment about that, but among these interviewees uncertainty related to screening and anxiety in receiving an indefinite result were clearly stated.

Religion was denied to be an important factor affecting decision-making although the **ethics** of abortion was a recognized factor by few women. In the latest case, the importance of ethical issues was correlated to invasive choice. Women were underlined how this aspect wasn't of such importance at screening stage, since pregnancy loss whether voluntary or spontaneous is not involved. **Parity** was indirectly indicated as another influencing factor, since normally knowledge searching was done at the first pregnancy and in subsequent once a pre-established pathway was followed (already mentioned "routine testing" for multiparous women). Finally one of the interviewees added that being a **single parent** versus having a partner's support made a big difference in decision-making, since taking on the risk of having a DS baby is then a sole responsibility with attendant consequences.

"…There were no factors to me to be honest…like you said nothing to do with ethical religion…anything like that…perhaps maybe your age or if you already have children…if you are a single parent or not…if you have got support…you know…then again it's difficult to bring up some children in this society nowadays…so that is one factor I would say…" (Multiparous, 21 yrs)

Chapter 4: Discussion & Conclusion

Knowledge and awareness of options varied greatly among women and the desire of making an informed decision was inconstantly identified at the screening stage. Some women followed a predetermined pathway, a routine, looking for a more paternalistic approach by HP.

Women didn't find the decision of being screened difficult because they were pretty determined to check whether the baby was fine. The main reasons why women wanted to get tested were reassurance, to be prepared or to terminate in case of DS.

There was a major confusion among the different options available in the screening category, but the difficult decision remained deciding whether to go for further testing in high-risk cases. Such confusion was due to lack of information, particularly for women referred by GP or other Hospitals. Previous pregnancies seemed to impact on options understanding and information seeking.

Most women choosing the Combined/Integrated Test either followed a suggested pathway or wanted to be as sure as possible without taking the risk of invasive procedures. Triple and Quadruple choices were related to disinformation, unavailability of other options at specific Trusts or late access to service.

The real decision women felt they had to make was whether to go for further testing in case of a positive result and in fact knowledge need was generally perceived at that stage.

The majority of women preferred to postpone any thoughts about invasive procedures and termination to after-screening moment, to avoid anxiety. Most patients wouldn't either consider possible consequences of going through screening (i.e. getting a positive result) or to choose an invasive procedure in the first place.

Among women aware of the different options, the choice was made mainly by balancing different factors. Main concerns involved were: the risk of having a Down's baby and the risk of pregnancy loss either miscarriage or termination.

Clearly the more a woman was concerned about having a Down's baby, the more she would focus her choice on tests' accuracy level. In addition relevant factors mentioned by women who had experienced invasive tests were: emotional and physical discomfort related to procedures, ethical issues and people' judgment related to abortion.

Although women would prefer to get earlier results, when they were asked to weight GA at tests/results & accuracy level they argued that a more accurate test even getting late results would be preferable. If some women considered prenatal decision a private matter, the other half appreciated supportive help by family, friends or HP.

The aim of this study was identifying decision-making characteristics to inform development of a DSS and to respond to an expressed need. In fact different studies were implemented to test new interventions to improve knowledge, but very few to develop intervention to aid women in their decision-making process (Green JM et al, 2004; Nagle C et al., 2007).

Previous work demonstrated an existing gap between women's willing to make an informed choice and their actual skills to do it (Green JM et al, 2004) and wish of being supported in thinking more deeply about factors affecting this choice (Santalahti P et al., 1998). Other strength of this project was the comprehensive approach to evaluate different factors involved in the decision, giving an overall picture of what a woman would go through.

Most of last years work focused on specific aspects of decision: some studies looking at theoretical models to explain women's decision and predict behaviors (Michie S et al., 2004; Bekker HL et al., 2004; Lumley MA et al., 2006; Van den Berg et al., 2008) others describing the impact of specific factors on decision-making (Etchegary H et al., 2008; Garcia E et al., 2008a; Van den Berg M et al., 2007; Garcia E et al., 2008b). This strength to be as comprehensive as possible represents also a weakness since we lost depth into single factors, to prioritize completeness.

Other weakness is related to sample demographic characteristics. In fact women accepting to participate were essentially Caucasian or Black and only two Asian women were included despite the recognized disparity in prenatal test participation among these ethnic groups (Fransen MP et al., 2007; Rowe et al., 2004).

Other limitation was deciding to interview women with their partners, if it was their desire. This could have influenced women in disclosing information, especially regarding the role of their partner in decision-making and how they felt about it.

As already recognized in previous research, this study showed how women were interested in acknowledging their baby's wellbeing (Garcia E et al., 2008 a) and how they perceived screening as a harmless, free and sensitive choice to ascertain this. As Green et al. reported screening was positively perceived by 75% of women recognizing it as a useful instrument to empower them, enabling them to make choices about their pregnancy (Green et al., 2004).

Knowledge and understanding of the difference between screening and diagnostic tests and risk attached was widely diffused. What women weren't clear about was the difference amongst tests belonging to those categories and how screening cut-off is arbitrary established. This is in contrast with previous research work reporting lack of knowledge even on the basic characteristics of screening (Green JM et al, 2004).

The reason why our interviewees' knowledge of basic principles was substantial could be related to experience, since 12 out of 20 were multiparous or maternal age since our sample's mean was over 35. Older age could enhance risk perception, affecting their search for knowledge.

This hypothesis is controversial though because women's perception of risk is not only related to biomedical definition of risky age but, to a certain extent, also to their lifestyle and how they physically feel (Lippman, 1999). To confirm the latest finding, in our study some women showed confidence in negativity of results because of their healthy lifestyle.

In line with previous work were reasons given by women to undertake DS tests: as part of routine care, to be reassured, to be prepared or to terminate pregnancy in case of DS (Green JM et al, 2004).

Few deviant cases reported as reasons obeying to doctor, age or family history of abnormalities. Latest cases confirmed the already proposed hypothesis that experiential knowledge would affect prenatal screening decisions (Etchegary et al., 2008). Obeying the doctor was the answer of a couple from an ethnical minority group and it could reflect a singular doctor-patient relationship due to different cultural context.

Depending on women's awareness, decision-making could be an informed weighing of values and preferences related to different options or simply following a predetermined pathway until screening results were received. Very few women had thought about possible outcomes of screening and most of them consciously avoid considering invasive options and TOP from the beginning.

Also these findings confirmed previous work: screening decisions are not predictive of either invasive procedure uptake or termination choices even though the same patterns of factors were identified as involved in diagnostic decision (Green et al., 2004).

In fact, prenatal decision about DS involves more than one decision for women. The first one about whether they want to be screened or not and which kind of tests they would prefer. The second one is about diagnostic procedure and eventual termination, if they were at high risk.

Because of that screening was mostly considered as a routine procedure, but the difficulties were identified at diagnostic even among women who didn't undertake invasive at current pregnancy. This is also the reason why more information was needed before invasive testing.
In terms of factors involved in decision-making our results mainly confirmed previous findings. Having a DS baby and spontaneous or voluntary pregnancy loss are crucial concerns of women making the decision. Attitude towards abortion is a very powerful predictor of testing decisions (Etchegary et al., 2008), so surely an important concern.

Attitude towards abortion is the best single predictor of invasive tests uptake, better than both actual and perceived risk (Tercyak et al., 2001). In consideration of our findings, confirmed by previous literature these factors were incorporated into our DSS[7].

The choice of distinguishing between first and second trimester TOP and miscarriage in our DSS was related to women's identification of timing as an issue involved in the decision among different tests. In our study as in previous work, women clearly stated that getting earlier results would be preferable to have time to decide for further steps (Ellis SM et al., 2006). Although when asked to balance accuracy and time, accuracy resulted the option of preference among our interviewees.

Emotional and physical discomfort related to invasive tests and anxiety related to uncertain results were mentioned as important concerns. These findings implied not only the inclusion of these factors as concerns into our DSS, but also reinforced the hypothesis of emotions as an essential component of decision.

---

[7] See Figure 2: DSS Annalisa & Down's syndrome Prenatal Choice

The importance of decisions' emotional aspect was expressed as a desire for new strategies to enhance emotional support. These are important elements against simplistic rational theories to explain prenatal decision. Decision-making is not merely based on rational or emotional modes but it's a very complex process involving multiple types of thinking and using these in the context of personal and professional relationships (Anderson G, 2007).

The last important explored aspect of decision-making was how people weight their concerns. How much a single individual is concerned about these outcomes derives from personal preferences. Those could be affected by ethics and subjective norms but not by religion, following our women's opinion.

Past literature looking at religiosity and ethical issues influence on prenatal decision-making is quite controversial. Among our interviewees religiosity wasn't mentioned as a factor affecting women's decision-making as Lumley et al. suggested (Lumley MA et al., 2006) but other authors supported this (Ahmed et al., 2006). This difference could be explained by ethnic groups variation affecting overall studies' results. Ethical beliefs were identified as a factor affecting decision among our women confirming other recent work (Garcia et al., 2008 a: Van den Berg et al., 2008).

Half of our women recognized prenatal decision as a private matter to be decided as a couple, the other half appreciated support either by family, friends' network or HP. Most women declared to have taken the decision with their partner, and whenever they talked about a private matter their partner was considered as part of it.

This finding is in contrast to a recent study which looked at couples' decision about screening and reporting women deciding about testing without discussing with their partner (Gottfresdttir H, 2007), but in line with Garcia et al. supporting the hypothesis that the partner is considered an intrinsic element of the decision-making process (Garcia et al., 2008).

In reality, their partners accompanied fifteen out of twenty women at the interviews and this peculiarity could have affected the reliability of our findings on this matter. Women could have been influenced by partners' presence, not feeling comfortable in disclosing different opinions about couple dynamics in taking prenatal decisions.

If a partner was identified as part of this microcosm, friends and family were considered more as an emotional support or a useful help in searching for information (Santalahti et al., 1998; Garcia et al., 2008 b), but the external world could also be seen as source of judgments by women going for invasive options.

Some women were more orientated to search for information and make an informed autonomous decision. In this case they conceptualized HP' role as a neutral provision of information about risk and impact of disability on child and family (Garcia et al., 2008b).

On the other hand some interviewees struggled in the decision process and they were expecting help by experts (Van den Berg M et al., 2007). In previous studies though, subjective norm of HP is a poor predictor of screening uptake (Minchie S et al., 2004).

The role of subjective norms and the impact of other's opinion on women's final decision were variable and women's perception was not necessarily hostile. Garcia et al. supported the hypothesis that autonomous decisions could be made even taking into account social influences on women's choice (Garcia et al., 2008).

Other authors recently affirmed how a shared decision-making approach, involving both clinician and patient, could be the most applicable method in this context (Hunt LM et al., 2004).

A miscellaneous of personal values, ethics and external characters' opinions seemed to affect how women would balance their main concerns in making decisions. We know that the prospect of different situations or outcomes vary widely between women e.g. anxiety due to not knowing baby's status or loosing a normal baby through miscarriage (Kuppermann et al, 2003).

Each woman gives different value to these factors and this is the reason why decisions about prenatal screening should be individualized on single user's values and a DSS could be helpful.

It wasn't really clear whether all women really wanted to take autonomous decisions at a screening stage though. Finding that some women didn't collect information about screening and follow routinely what was offered to them could be a clear sign that they didn't want to take responsibility of making an informed choice.

However it was a completely different story when it came to decide about invasive procedure, because of the risk of miscarriage and possible termination. Knowledge demand increased at the diagnostic stage and it could be an expression of willingness to make decisions.

Desire to make an autonomous decision about prenatal screening and level of knowledge could be related. Explorative research into how attitudes towards having a DS child and abortion would affect willing to making an informed decision and knowledge searching is needed.

An assessment of whether women are willing to make an independent choice is related to diagnostic stage but not to screening is also needed. The best source of information about decision-making seemed to be nulliparous women, since most of the time once a woman/couple has searched for information in her first pregnancy, she tends to follow the same direction for the following.

Despite the general aim to move away from paternalistic approach to health decisions, the actual routinely acceptance of the majority of women of a screening test doesn't demonstrate a big change in such method. Green et al. suggested new interventions implementation to support women's decision-making (Green et al., 2004).

According to our women, rationality and emotions were both components of the decision and emotional support was suggested as a future improvement in Down's ANC. Empirical evidence on how decision aids would positively affect both cognitive and emotional mechanisms in prenatal counseling was collected in a recent RCT carried out in the UK (Bekker et al., 2003) and these findings would support a wider application of decision aids in this context.

If our starting point was that not all women really aimed to make an informed choice at the screening stage and that individuality of decision-making should be respected, then the use of DSS would be worth supporting exclusively diagnostic choices. Before undertaking diagnostic tests the use of a DSS would help enhancing knowledge and awareness that was recognized as a need at that stage by women.

At the screening stage, since not all women like to make decisions, the routine use of a DSS could increase anxiety and push women to make decisions they may not want to make, leading to ethical concerns and doubts about respect of individuality in decision-making. Furthermore it would mean to concretely collapse screening, diagnostic and termination decisions in one only and on the base of our findings this doesn't apply to women's decision-making reality.

On the other hand if women could be aware from the beginning of the consequences of a positive screening results focusing on what they really wanted, resources could be saved e.g. women willing to be 100% sure could undertake directly an invasive procedure without requiring a screening test first. Furthermore the emotional shock and pressure felt to decide in few days about diagnostic decisions would be solved, since women should start thinking of what could happen at 8 weeks.

Use of a DSS would respect individuality of single woman's values and could enhance awareness offering the possibility of moving a step further towards autonomous prenatal choices. Giving for true that most women appreciated a paternalistic approach at screening stage, it would be necessary to balance ethical issues related to pushing women to make choices they might not want to make at that stage and the economical and emotional advantages derived from stimulating a conscious, autonomous and informed choice.

References

1.   Ahmed S, Atkin K, Hewison J, Green J. The influence of faith and religion and the role of religious and community leaders in prenatal decisions for sickle cell disorders and thalassaemia major. Prenat Diagn 2006; 26: 801-809.

2.   Anderson G. Patient decision-making for clinical genetics. Nursing Inquiry 2007; 14(1): 13-22.

3.   Bekker H, Thornton JG, Airey CM, Connelly JB, Hewison J, Robinson MB, Lilleyman J, MacIntosh M, Maule AJ, Michie S, Pearman AD. Informed decision-making: an annotated bibliography and systematic review. Health Technology Assessment 1999; 3: No 1.

4.   Bekker H, Hewison J, Thorton JG. Understanding why decision aids work: linking process with outcome. Patient Education and Counselling 2003; 50: 323-329.

5.   Bekker H, Hewison J, Thorthon JG. Applying decision analysis to facilitate informed decision making about prenatal diagnosis for Down syndrome: a randomized control trial. Prenat Diagn 2004; 24:265-275.

6.   Benn P. Improved antenatal screening for Down's syndrome. The Lancet 2003; 361(9360):794-5.

7.   Copel JA, Bahado-Singh RO. Prenatal Screening for Down's syndrome – a search for the family's values (Editorial). N.Engl.J.Med. 1999; 341: 521-2.

8.   Etchegary H, Potter B, Howley H, Cappelli M, Coyle D, Graham I, Walker M, Wilson B. The influence of Experiential Knowledge on Prenatal Screening and Testing Decisions.   Genetic Testing 2008; 12(1):115-124.

9.   Fransen MP, Essink-Bot ML, Oenema A, Mackenbach JP, Steegers EAP, Wildschut HIJ. Ethnic differences in determinants of participation and non-participation in prenatal screening for Down's syndrome: A theoretical framework. Prenat Diagn 2007; 27:938-950.

10.   French R, Dowie J. Using decision analysis to help young people with contraceptive choices. In Teenage Pregnancy and Reproductive Health. Eds. Baker P, Guthrie K, Hutchinson C, Kane R and Wellings K. 2007 RCOG Press, London.

11.   Garcia E, Timmermans DRM, van Leeuwen E. The impact of ethical beliefs on decisions about prenatal screening tests: Searching for justification. Social Science & Medicine 2008: 66:753-764. (a)

12.   Garcia E, Timmermans DRM, van Leeuwen E. Rethinking autonomy in the context of prenatal screening decision-making. Prenat Diagn 2008; 28:115-120. (b)

13.   Green JM, Hewison J, Bekker HL, Bryant LD, Cockle HS. Psychosocial aspects of genetic screening of pregnant women and newborns: a systematic review. Health Technology Assessment 2004; 8, No. 33.

14.   Gottfredsdottir H, Sandall J, Bjornsdottir K. "This is just what you do when you are pregnant": a qualitative study of prospective parents in Iceland who accept nuchal translucency screening. Midwifery 2008; doi: 10.1016/j.midw.2007.12.004.

15.   Gorounti K, Sandall J. Do pregnant women in Greece make informed choices about antenatal screening for Down's syndrome? A questionnaire survey. Midwifery 2008; 24:153-162.

16.   Haddow J, Palomaki GE, Knight GJ, Cunningham GC, Lustig LS, Boyd PA. Reducing the need for amniocentesis in women 35 years old of age or older with serum markers for screening. N.Engl.J.Med.1994; 330:1114-8.

17.   Hall S, Bobrow M, Marteau TM. Psychological consequences for parents of false negative results on prenatal screening for Down's syndrome: retrospective interview study. Br.Med.J. 2000; 320:407-12.

18.   Hunt LM, de Voogd KB, Castaneda H. The routine and the traumatic in prenatal genetic diagnosis: does clinical information inform patient decision-making? Patient Education and Counselling 2005; 56: 302-312.

19.   Kuppermann M, Nease Jr RF, Harris R, Washington AE. Cost utility of prenatal diagnosis (letter). The Lancet 2003; 363:1165.

20.   Lewis SM, Cullinane FM, Carlin JB, Halliday JL. Women's and health professionals' preferences for prenatal testing for Down's syndrome in Australia. Australian and New Zealand Journal of Obstetrics and Gynaecology 2006; 46: 205-211.

21.   Lippman A. Embodied knowledge and making sense of prenatal diagnosis. J Genet Couns 8:255-273.

22.   Lumley MA, Zamerowski ST, Jackson L, Dukes K, Sullivan L. Psychosocial correlates of Pregnant Women's attitudes toward Prenatal Maternal Serum Screening and Invasive Diagnostic Testing: Beyond Traditional Risk Status. Genetic Testing 2006; 10(2): 131-138.

23.   Marteau T, Dormandy E, Minchie S. A measure of informed choice. Health Expectations 2001; 4:99-108.

24.   Minchie S, Dormandy E, French DP, Marteu T. Using theory of planned behaviour to predict screening uptake in two contexts. Psychology and Health 2004; 19(6): 705-718.

25.   Nagle C, Gunn J, Bell R, Lewis S, Meiser B, Metcalfe S, Ukoumunne OC, Halliday J. Use of a decision aid for prenatal testing of fetal abnormalities to improve women's informed decision making: a cluster randomized controlled trial [ISRCTN22532458]. BJOG 2008; 115:339-347.

26.   National Collaborating Centre for Women's and Children's Health. Antenatal Care: routine care for healthy pregnant woman. Clinical Guideline March 2008. RCOG Press, London.

27.   Rowe RE, Garcia J, Davidson LL. Social and ethnic inequalities in the offer and uptake of prenatal screening and diagnosis in the UK: a systematic review. Public Health 2004; 118:177-189.

28.   Royal College of Obstetricians and Gynaecologists. Amniocentesis and Chorionic Villous Sampling. Guideline No. 8. January 2005.

29.   Santalahti P, Hemminki E, Latikka AM, Ryynanen M. Women's Decision-making in prenatal screening. Soc. Sci. Med. 1998; 8: 1067-1076.

30.   Stone DH, Rosenberg K, Womersley J. Recent trends in the prevalence and secondary prevention of Down's syndrome. Paediatric and Perinatal Epidemiology 1989; 3(3): 278-283.

31.   Tercyak KP, Bennet Johnson S, Roberts SF, Cruz AC. Psychological response to prenatal genetic counselling and amniocentesis. Patient Education Counselling 2001; 43: 73-84.

32.   Van den Berg M, Timmermans DRM, Kleinveld JH, van Eijk JTM, Knol DL, van der Wal G, van Vugt JMG. Are counsellors' attitudes influencing pregnant women's attitudes and decisions on prenatal screening? Prenat Diagn 2007; 27:518-524.

33.   Van den Berg M, Timmermans DRM, Knol DL, De Smit DJ, Van Eijk JTM, Van Vugt JMG, Van der Wal G. Understanding Pregnant Women's Decision Making Concerning Prenatal Screening. Health Psychology 2008; 27(4):430-437.

34.   Wald NJ, Rodeck C, Hackshaw AK, Walters J, Chitty L, Mackinson AM et al. First and second trimester antenatal screening for Down's syndrome: the results of the Serum, Urine and Ultrasound Screening Study (SURUSS). Health Technology Assessment 2003; 7:1-77.

Appendix

ANC	Antenatal care
AFP	Alpha-fetoprotein
CVS	Chorionic villous sampling
DR	Detection Rate
DS	Down's syndrome
DSS	Decision support system
EDD	Expected date at delivery
FPR	False Positive Rate
GA	Gestational age
GP	General practitioner
β-hCG	Free β Human chorionic gonadotrophin
HP	Health Professionals
MCDA	Multi-criteria Decision Models
NCC-WCH	National collaborating centre for Women's and Children's Health
NT	Nuchal translucency
PAPP-A	Pregnancy-associated plasma protein-A
RCT	Randomized control trial
R, I, P	Respondent, Interviewer, Partner
RCOG	Royal College of Obstetricians & Gynecologists
SEU	Subjective Expected Utility
TOP	Termination of pregnancy
uE3	Unconjugated estriol

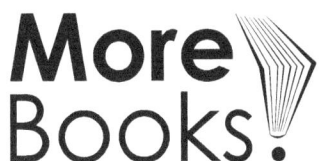
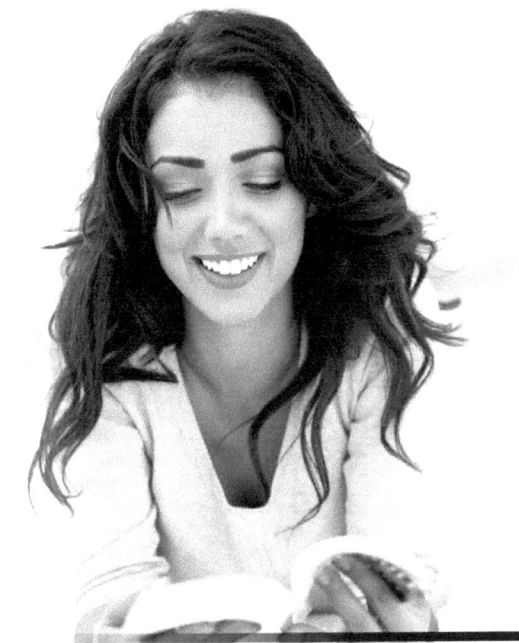
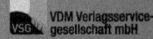

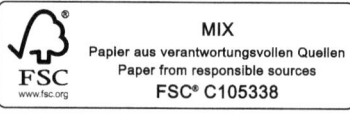